The Ultimate Cabbage Soup Diet

The Ultimate Cabbage Soup Diet

MADELINE COOPER

JOHN BLAKE

Published by John Blake Publishing Ltd,
3, Bramber Court, 2 Bramber Road,
London W14 9PB, England

This edition published in paperback in 2003

ISBN 1 904034 84 5

This book has been previously published as
The Cabbage Soup Diet Recipe Book.

British Library Cataloguing-in-Publication Data:

A catalogue record for this book is
available from the British Library.

Design by ENVY

Printed in Great Britain by Bookmarque

1 3 5 7 9 10 8 6 4 2

Papers used by John Blake Publishing are natural, recyclable products made
from wood grown in sustainable forests. The manufacturing processes
conform to the environmental regulations of the country of origin.

Contents

Introduction

Introduction

It is important that you read this introduction. It contains all the details of the Cabbage Soup Diet, as well as a few rules that you must follow.

Congratulations! You have chosen the Cabbage Soup Diet because it's the fastest weight-loss programme around. It takes just a week, and most people lose up to ten pounds in that time. Sounds incredible? Well, it *is* incredible – but it's also true.

The purpose of this book is to show you a hundred ways of making the diet not just a week of slog, but something you'll actually look forward to. You'll probably even find that you'll want to use some of these recipes when you're not even on the diet. They are all healthy, very low in fat – and delicious.

Before we start on the recipes themselves, there are a few important things you need to know. We'll explain how to use the Cabbage Soup Diet and exactly what you can eat on each of the seven days. Then we'll explain how to use this book, before going over a few rules that you must abide by. But

3

first, we'll answer the question everybody wants to know: *Why is the Cabbage Soup Diet so popular?*

1. **It really works.** The Cabbage Soup Diet is *not* just another fad diet. Men and women across the world have had incredible success with this diet, making it one of the most popular in history.
2. **It's quick.** The diet only takes seven days, after which time you can revert to your normal eating patterns.
3. **You never feel hungry.** This is at the centre of the diet's popularity. On each day, you can eat as much as you like of certain foods, so you don't have to suffer the misery of an empty tummy!

The Cabbage Soup Diet is really, really easy to follow. In a nutshell, it lasts for seven days, and on each day you are allowed as much as you like of a very nutritious, very tasty soup. In addition, on certain days you are allowed unlimited quatitites of what are known as 'free' fruits and vegetables. You will find a list of these 'free' fruits and vegetables later on in this introduction. On one day you can eat a jacket potato, on another day lots of bananas. And on each day you are allowed a limited quantity of either skimmed milk or low-fat yoghurt. Essentially that's all there is to it. Simple isn't it? Let's have a look at the actual diet.

The Cabbage Soup Diet

This is a day-by-day list of exactly what you can eat on each day of the diet:

Day 1
- Cabbage Soup
- Unlimited free fruits
- 1x8fl oz serving skimmed milk or low-fat natural yoghurt
- Tea or coffee, plain, or with artificial sweetener
- 1 tbsp low- or no-fat salad dressing

Day 2
- Cabbage Soup
- Unlimited free vegetables
- 1 large baked potato
- 1 8fl oz serving skimmed milk or low-fat natural yoghurt
- Tea or coffee, plain, or with artificial sweetener
- 1 tbsp low- or no-fat salad dressing

Day 3

- Cabbage Soup
- Unlimited free vegetables
- Unlimited free fruits
- 1x8fl oz serving skimmed milk or low-fat natural yoghurt
- Tea or coffee, plain, or with artificial sweetener
- 1 tbsp low- or no-fat salad dressing

Day 4

- Cabbage Soup
- 3-6 bananas
- 8x8fl oz glasses skimmed milk, or 1x8fl oz serving plain, low-fat natural yoghurt and 7x8fl oz glasses skimmed milk

Day 5

- Cabbage Soup
- Unlimited fish
- Unlimited chicken
- Up to six tomatoes
- 1x8fl oz serving skimmed milk or low-fat natural yoghurt
- Tea or coffee, plain, or with artificial sweetener
- 1 tbsp low- or no-fat salad dressing

Day 6
- Cabbage Soup
- Unlimited fish
- Unlimited chicken
- Unlimited free vegetables, including tomatoes
- 1x8fl oz serving skimmed milk or low-fat natural yoghurt
- Tea or coffee, plain, or with artificial sweetener
- 1 tbsp low- or no-fat salad dressing

Day 7
- Cabbage Soup
- Unlimited free vegetables
- Unlimited free fruits
- 1x8oz serving skimmed milk or low-fat natural yoghurt
- Tea or coffee, plain, or with artificial sweetener
- 1 tbsp low- or no-fat salad dressing

It really is as simple as that!

What are Free Fruit and Vegetables?

Free Vegetables

Artichokes

Asparagus

Aubergine

Beans

Beetroot

Broccoli

Brussels Sprouts

Cabbage

Carrots

Cauliflower

Celery

Courgettes

Cucumber

Greens, leafy (Spinach, Endive, Chicory, Sorrel)

Lettuces

Mushrooms

Onions

Parsley

Peppers

Radishes

Turnips

Free Fruits

Apples

Apricots

Berries

Blueberries

Cherries

Grapefruit

Grapes

Kiwi Fruit

Lemons

Melons

Nectarines

Oranges

Peaches

Pineapple

Plums

Strawberries

Tangerines

* Tomatoes are *not* free vegetables, but you are allowed a limited number of tomatoes on day 5, and an unlimited number on day 6.

INTRODUCTION

In addition, and here is where this book really comes into its own, you are allowed to flavour your food with just about any no- or low-calorie ingredient you choose. This includes fresh or dried herbs, spices, hot sauces, soy sauce, vinegars, ketchup, lemon juice – you'll find all these things used to great effect here.

You will also see that, although sugar is obviously taboo, you *can* use low-calorie sweetener. We've tried to keep this to a minimum, but if you need a bit of sweetness, go ahead and use a low-calorie sweetener.

Important

You are only allowed to have *either* 8fl oz low-fat yoghurt *or* 8fl oz skimmed milk on each day. This means that if you eat 5fl oz of low-fat yoghurt for breakfast, then you cannot have any skimmed milk on that day, but you *must* have a further 3fl oz low-fat yoghurt to make up your daily allowance. Or if you choose to have 2fl oz skimmed milk for lunch on day 2, then you must have a further 6fl oz skimmed milk later in the day – but *no* low-fat yoghurt. Use the relevant boxes in the Ingredients Table at the back of the book to keep track of your daily intake. The exception to this is on day 4, when you are allowed to substitute *one* of the 8x8fl oz skimmed milk with 1x8fl oz low-fat yoghurt.

How to Use This Book

As you can see, the possibilities are almost endless. On some days you can eat as much fish or chicken as you want; on other days you can eat your fill of vegetables and fruit. There are all sorts of combinations. But anybody is going to get bored of eating just plain fish or plain vegetables. Maybe you are too busy to devise interesting menus for your weekly diet; perhaps you need to incorporate certain dishes into your family's menu so that you can diet without being the odd one out; or maybe you just want a little bit of inspiration. That's where this book comes in.

In the pages of this book, you will find a hundred recipes that can be used as part of the diet. Of course, you can't use the recipes randomly – certain dishes are only allowed on certain days – but if you look at each recipe you will see something that looks like this:

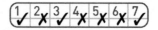

The numbers that are ticked mean that you can eat this particular recipe on that day of the diet. The numbers that are crossed indicate the days on which the recipe is not allowed. In this instance, you could eat the recipe on days 1, 3 and 7; but not on days 2, 4, 5 or 6.

The Ingredients Table

On pages 188-9, you will find an ingredients table. You can photocopy this if you like, and use it each time you do the diet. On this table, you must tick off each restricted ingredient as you use it. That way, you will be able to keep track of what you must and must not eat. This is important – if, on day 2, for example, you have a breakfast that involves 8fl oz of low-fat yoghurt, you can't have another meal that day that includes yoghurt. By ticking off your yoghurt allowance on the ingredients table, you can easily avoid making a mistake.

A Few Rules Before You Start

As you can see, the Cabbage Soup Diet is not difficult. But it *is* strict, and there are a few rules that you must abide by if you want to lose weight successfully.

1.   Check with your doctor before starting this diet. The Cabbage Soup Diet is suitable for most people, with the exception of children or adolescents, but as

it is such a fast weight-loss regime, certain medical conditions may make it unsuitable for you. Do check.

2. Make sure you eat at least two portions of cabbage soup every day. This is important because it contains lots of nutrients to keep you going through the week. If you get bored of the original Cabbage Soup, there are a few suggestions in the Soups section on how to spice it up.

3. Don't omit foods. Everything on the diet is there for a reason. As we have said, the cabbage soup itself is very nutritious. Similarly, the free fruits and vegetables contain essential nutrients and fibre. The chicken and fish on days 5 and 6 help to boost the protein content of the diet, so you should try and eat at least one chicken dish and one fish dish on each of those days. And all those bananas on day 4 are there to provide you with Vitamin A, niacin, iron, some protein and plenty of potassium. All these elements make the diet well balanced and healthy. Don't skip them!

4. Although you are allowed unlimited quantities of certain foods, don't go mad! Eat until you feel

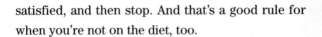

satisfied, and then stop. And that's a good rule for when you're not on the diet, too.

5. No alcohol.

6. When cooking chicken, do remove all the skin. This is easy to do, and will make all the difference as the skin contains all the fat that we want to avoid.

7. On each day you are allowed *either* skimmed milk *or* low-fat natural yoghurt. **You are not allowed to mix the two.** So if you start a particular day with a recipe involving 4fl oz low-fat yoghurt, you cannot drink any milk on that day. The only exception to this rule is on day 4, when you are allowed to replace one of your 8x8fl oz of skimmed milk with an 8fl oz serving of low-fat yoghurt.

8. Don't use flavourings or condiments that contain more than 25 calories per tablespoon.

9. Do remember that, although you can eat unlimited quantities of certain ingredients on particular days, this does not mean that you can eat unlimited quantities of all of these recipes, as they may also contain ingredients that are restricted on that

particular day. Use the ingredients table at the back of the book to monitor how much of each ingredient you have consumed.

10. This is seven-day plan which induces intensive weight-loss **and should therefore not be used for longer than a one-week period.** You must then have a break of *at least two weeks* before using it again.

A Few Culinary Tips

1.   Don't be afraid to have food for breakfast that you wouldn't normally think of. Soup or fish for breakfast is a really good way of setting you up for the day.

2.   In quite a few recipes, you will see that you are required to cook vegetables in the microwave. You will not find detailed instruction on how to do this in the book, as it will vary from machine to machine. Check your manufacturer's instructions for the cooking of vegetables if you are unsure how to go about it.

3.   Don't be surprised that lemon juice is used on non-free fruit days. It's just the juice, and is very low-calorie. It's fine to use it as a flavouring.

4. Most of the recipes in the book are for one person. Some are for more. You can increase or decrease the number of people you're cooking for simply by doubling or halving the quantities involved. **If you do this, make sure you keep track of the amount of restricted ingredients you yourself are eating. Remember that you can use the ingredients table at the back of the book to do this.**

That's it! You now know everything you need to embark upon this incredible diet. Enjoy, good luck and watch the weight drop off!

Basics

Basics

Throughout this book, you will find certain ingredients called for on a number of occasions. The first, naturally, is cabbage soup. You'll be eating this every day for a week, so it makes sense to cook up a large amount, and then keep it in the fridge or freeze it. The recipe given here makes about 12 pints.

Because the diet doesn't allow the use of oil or butter, we will have to use other ways of cooking. Poaching vegetables, fish or chicken in stock is a very good way of doing this, and you'll find that a number of recipes call for either vegetable or fish stock – particularly vegetable. Again, it would be a good idea to prepare a supply of this at the beginning of your week, and then keep it in the fridge or freeze it in small quantities, whichever you prefer. And remember, these stocks will come in handy, even when you're not on the diet!

The Original Cabbage Soup

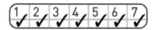

Don't forget that you can eat this hot or cold; and look in the Soups section for some great variations.

Makes about 12 pints

1 cabbage
6 carrots
6 medium onions
6 spring onions
2 green or red peppers, de-seeded
3 large tomatoes
5 stalks celery, trimmed
4oz (110g) uncooked brown rice
salt and freshly-ground black pepper

Cut the vegetables into bite-sized pieces. Place in a large, 12-pint pot and add enough cold water to cover. Bring to the boil, and then simmer uncovered for about 10 minutes. Cover, and then simmer on a low heat until the vegetables are soft. This should take about an hour. Whilst the soup is simmering, cook the rice according to the instructions on the packet. When the soup is almost cooked, add the rice, and then season to taste with the salt and pepper. Allow to cool, and then keep in the fridge, or freeze – whichever is most convenient.

Vegetable Stock

This will make 5-6 pints, but it would be a good idea to freeze it in small quantities to use as required.

1 lb (450g) carrots
1 lb (450g) onions
half a head of celery
1 small piece of turnip
1 bouquet garni
a few black peppercorns
1 level dsp salt
6 pints (3.5l) boiling water

Peel and wash the vegetables, slice into big pieces, and then place in a large pan with the boiling water and the rest of the ingredients. Simmer, half-covered, for 3 hours, or until the stock has a good flavour. It should reduce by about a third. Strain, and use as required.

Fish Stock

Fish stock is called for in a few of the fish recipes, and is very easy to make.

Makes about 2 ½ pints

1¼lb (560g) bones from assorted white fish
1 onion
1 carrot
1 bouquet garni
6 black peppercorns
1 tsp salt
1 blade of mace
2½ pints (1.5l) water
juice of a lemon
1 strip of lemon peel

Wash the bones and break them into two or three pieces. Put into a pan with all the other ingredients. Bring to the boil, partly cover, and simmer for about 30 minutes. Strain off and cool.

Soups

Soups

Soup, of course, is the mainstay of the Cabbage Soup Diet. You'll be eating as much cabbage soup as you like, which means that you needn't feel hungry at any point throughout the week. In this section you will find four variations on the original cabbage soup, which you can eat on any day of the week.

You'll also find six other soup recipes. Remember that you can only eat these on the days specified. *You should eat cabbage soup on these days as well. These other soups would make a good starter on the days they're allowed, though, or a tasty mid-afternoon snack. Just remember to tick off any restricted ingredients you use on the ingredients table at the back of the book!*

Cabbage Soup Italiano

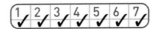

Makes about 12 pints

1 cabbage
6 carrots
6 medium onions
6 spring onions
2 green or red peppers, de-seeded
3 large tomatoes
5 stalks celery, trimmed
4oz (110g) uncooked brown rice
a few good handfuls flat-leaf parsley (to taste), chopped
3 cloves garlic, crushed
2 heaped tbsp fresh oregano leaves, crushed
1 tsp dried oregano
salt and freshly-ground black pepper

Cut the vegetables into bite-sized pieces. Place into a
large 12-pint pot, with the parsley, garlic, oregano, salt
and pepper, and then add enough cold water to cover.
Bring to the boil and allow to cook for 10 minutes.
Reduce the heat, cover, and allow to simmer gently until
the vegetables are soft. This should take about an hour.

Meanwhile, cook the rice according to the packet
instructions. When the soup is cooked, add the rice and
then season to taste.

TIP: If you don't want to make large quantities of Cabbage Soup
Italiano, you could just add the parsley, garlic and oregano in smaller
quantities to a bowl of the original soup.

Szechuan Cabbage Soup

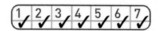

Makes about 12 pints

1 cabbage
6 carrots
6 medium onions
6 spring onions
2 green or red peppers, de-seeded
3 large tomatoes
5 stalks celery, trimmed
4oz (110g) uncooked brown rice
6-8 thinly-sliced spring onions
2-4 tbsp soy sauce
1 tsp Chinese chilli paste
salt and freshly-ground black pepper

Cut the vegetables into bite-sized pieces. Place into a large 12-pint pot, with the spring onions, soy sauce, chilli paste, salt and pepper, and then add enough cold water to cover. Bring to the boil and allow to cook for ten minutes. Reduce the heat, cover, and allow to simmer gently until the vegetables are soft.

TIP: If you don't want to make large quantities of Szechuan Cabbage Soup, you could just add the spring onions, soy sauce and chilli paste in smaller quantities to a bowl of the original soup.

This should take about an hour.

Meanwhile, cook the rice according to the packet instructions. When the soup is cooked, add the rice and then season to taste.

Bengal Cabbage Soup

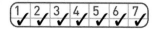

Makes about 12 pints

1 cabbage
6 carrots
6 medium onions
6 spring onions
2 green or red peppers, de-seeded
3 large tomatoes
5 stalks celery, trimmed
2 cucumbers, peeled and sliced
2 tsp ground cumin
2 tsp ground turmeric
a hint of saffron, if you have it
salt and freshly-ground black pepper

Cut the vegetables into bite-sized pieces. Place into a large 12-pint pot, with the cucumber, cumin, turmeric, saffron, salt and pepper, and then add enough cold water to cover. Bring to the boil and allow to cook for 10 minutes. Reduce the heat, cover, and allow to simmer gently until the vegetables are soft. This should take about an hour.

> TIP: If you don't want to make large quantities of Bengal Cabbage Soup, you could just add the cucumber, cumin, turmeric and saffron in smaller quantities to a bowl of the original soup.

Meanwhile, cook the rice according to the packet instructions. When the soup is cooked, add the rice and then season to taste.

Cauliflower Soup

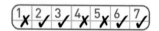

Serves 2

the white part of 1 small cauliflower
12fl oz (330ml) vegetable stock
8fl oz (220ml) skimmed milk
salt and freshly-ground black pepper
a little grated nutmeg
a few chives, chopped

Chop the cauliflower into florets and cook in the boiling vegetable stock for 12-15 minutes until tender. Liquidise the cauliflower and stock in a food processor. Put the milk in a pan, add the cauliflower purée, season with salt, pepper and a little nutmeg, and heat through. Garnish with the chives and serve.

Greek Plaki (Fish Soup)

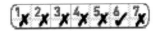

This is a hearty, casserole-type soup which is very filling and delicious.

Serves 2

1½lb (700g) assorted white fish fillet
salt and freshly-ground black pepper
1½ tbsp lemon juice
2 large onions, sliced
2 garlic cloves, crushed
2 tbsp parsley, chopped
4oz (110g) tomatoes, skinned, de-seeded and chopped
8fl oz (220g) water
rind and juice of 2 lemons
2 extra lemons, sliced
2 extra tomatoes, sliced

Trim the fillets, wash and wipe dry, season with salt and pepper and sprinkle with the lemon juice. Cook the onion and garlic in the microwave, until soft. Transfer to a pan, add the tomatoes and water, and simmer until the tomatoes are soft. Put in the fish, making sure it is well impregnated with the pan juices, garnish with the slices of lemon and tomato, cover, simmer for 20 minutes, and serve.

Mushroom Soup

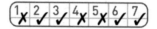

Young field mushrooms, with pale brown gills, are best for this soup. Older mushrooms with blackened gills give a good flavour but make the soup very dark.

Serves 2

4oz (110g) mushrooms
6fl oz skimmed milk
2 tbsp lemon juice
1 tbsp parsley, chopped

Set aside 1 or 2 small mushrooms for garnishing. Chop the remainder and cook gently in the lemon juice until tender. Purée the mushrooms in a liquidiser, keeping them quite coarse, as this gives the soup a more interesting texture. Strain the juice from the mushrooms and make it up to 7½fl oz (210ml) with the milk. Add the mushrooms to the liquid, season with salt and pepper, bring slowly to the boil and simmer for 2-3 minutes. Sprinkle with chopped parsley, and a few sliced raw mushrooms.

Cucumber and Mint Soup

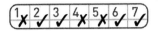

This is a delicious cold soup, ideal for hot sunny days!

Serves 1

1 medium-sized, firm, young cucumber
4fl oz (110ml) low-fat natural yoghurt
1 small clove garlic, crushed
1 tsp lemon juice
1 tsp fresh garden mint, chopped
a few slices lemon, cut very thinly
salt and freshly-ground black pepper

Peel the cucumber thinly, leaving a little of the green, then slice it. Keep a few thinly-cut slices as a garnish. Place the rest in a liquidiser with the yoghurt and crushed garlic. Blend until the mixture is smooth. Add the salt, pepper and lemon juice. If the soup appears to be too thick at this stage, you can thin it with some vegetable stock. Stir in the chopped mint, cover and chill for a few hours. Serve with the slices of cucumber and lemon on each portion.

Asparagus Soup

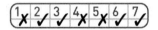

Serves 4

30 medium-sized heads of asparagus
1 shallot
1½ pints (850ml) vegetable stock
salt and pepper
1 tbsp parsley, chopped

Wash and trim the asparagus, lightly scraping the white part of the stalks and reserving about 6 of the smaller tips for a garnish. Cut the stalks into 1-inch lengths, and slice the shallot finely. Put together in a pan with the stock. Cover and simmer for 30 minutes.

Meanwhile, blanch the reserved tips by placing them in cold water and bringing to the boil, refresh, and then cook in water until just tender. The preliminary blanching will keep them green.

Put the soup into a liquidiser. When liquidised, reheat and add parsley and seasoning. Serve in a bowl, and float the reserved tips on the top.

If you like, you can add a dessertspoon of low-fat yoghurt, but remember to subtract this from your daily allowance – and if you have yoghurt, remember you cannot have any milk on this day!

Tomato and Sorrel Soup

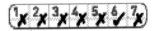

Sorrel is a refreshing herb which has been used for hundreds of years. It is very easy to grow in the garden, but can sometimes be difficult to find in the shops. A delicious variation is to use watercress instead.

Serves 3-4

2-3oz (50-75g) sorrel or watercress leaves
1lb (450g) tomatoes
4oz (110g) shallots or spring onions, skinned and roughly chopped
1 pint (570ml) vegetable stock
1 tbsp lemon juice
1 tbsp fresh tarragon, chopped
salt and freshly-ground black pepper

Cut off the stems and wash the sorrel thoroughly. Drain well. Cut the tomatoes into quarters, and then place them with the onions in the microwave and cook until tender. Put the cooked vegetables into a pan with the vegetable stock, bring to the boil and simmer for 10 minutes. Liquidise in small batches, add the lemon juice, chopped tarragon, salt and pepper. This soup is equally good served hot or cold. If you are serving cold, you could float a cube of ice in the middle after refrigerating.

Tex-Mex Cabbage Soup

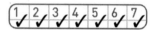

Makes about 12 pints

1 cabbage
6 carrots
6 medium onions
6 spring onions
2 green or red peppers, de-seeded
3 large whole tomatoes
5 stalks celery, trimmed
3-4 tsp chilli powder (either mild or strong)
4 jalapeno peppers, de-seeded and finely chopped
salt and pepper

Cut the vegetables into bite-sized pieces. Place into a large 12-pint pot, with the chilli powder, jalapeno peppers, salt and pepper, and then add enough cold water to cover. Bring to the boil and allow to cook for 10 minutes. Reduce the heat, cover, and allow to simmer gently until the vegetables are soft. This should take about an hour.

Meanwhile, cook the rice according to the packet instructions. When the soup is cooked, add the rice and then season to taste.

> TIP: If you don't want to make large quantities of Tex-Mex Cabbage Soup, you could just add the chilli powder and jalapeno peppers in smaller quantities to a bowl of the original soup.

Chicken
Dishes

Chicken Dishes

On days 5 and 6, you can eat as much chicken as you want. Do remember to remove the skin – not that you'll want it for any of these delicious recipes, all of them cooked in very low-fat ways.

Chicken en Papillotte

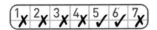

Dishes cooked en papillotte are wrapped in parchment paper or foil, then baked. This retains the moisture during cooking. If you're using this recipe on day 5, remember to deduct tomatoes from your allowance.

Serves 1

1x8oz (225g) breast of chicken, skin removed
4 tomatoes, sliced
1 dsp lemon juice
1 tsp fresh thyme, chopped
a few chives, chopped
a few basil leaves
1 tbsp low-calorie dressing
salt and freshly-ground black pepper

Pre-heat the oven to Gas Mark 5/190°C/375°F. Cut a square of parchment paper large enough to wrap around the chicken piece loosely. Take two of the sliced tomatoes and place them in the centre of the parchment. Season with salt and pepper. Place the chicken on top of the tomatoes, and sprinkle with lemon juice, thyme and chives. Wrap the parchment around the chicken, and scrunch up at the top so that no steam will escape. Place on a baking tray and bake for about 20 minutes, or until the chicken is cooked. Serve with a salad made of the remaining tomatoes, basil leaves, dressing, salt and pepper.

> TIP: This is an ideal recipe for day 5, but on day 6 you could also serve it with another vegetable dish.

Chicken and Tomato Kebabs

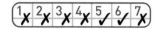

Skewering the kebabs on rosemary stalks infuses them with a lovely flavour. If you're using this recipe on day 5, remember to deduct the tomatoes from your tomato allowance – three cherry tomatoes are about the equivalent of 1 ordinary tomato.

Serves 1

8oz (225g) chicken breast, skin removed
8 cherry tomatoes
a few bay leaves, fresh if you have them
2 strong rosemary stalks, leaves removed (or kebab skewers)
2 ripe tomatoes
a few basil leaves
1 tbsp low-calorie dressing

For the Marinade
1 tbsp low-fat natural yoghurt
1 tsp lemon juice
salt and freshly-ground black pepper
½ tsp dried mixed herbs

Chop the chicken breast into bite-sized pieces. Mix the marinade ingredients together and then add the chicken. Put in the fridge for a couple of hours. Thread the chicken, cherry tomatoes and bay leaves on to the rosemary stalks or kebab skewers, and grill

TIP: This is an ideal recipe for day 5, but on day 6 you could also serve it with another vegetable dish.

until the chicken is cooked. In the meantime, slice the remaining tomatoes and make a salad with the dressing and the basil leaves. Serve the kebabs with the tomato salad.

Stuffed Breast of Chicken

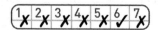

Serves 1

1x8oz (225g) chicken breast, skin removed
2fl oz (55ml) vegetable stock
1 tsp grated carrot
1 tsp chopped shallot
1 tsp chopped tarragon
1 tsp low-fat yoghurt

To serve
½ red onion, diced
½ green pepper, diced
a small piece turnip, diced
½ carrot, diced
½ stick celery, diced
1 tsp chopped parsley
a little vegetable stock to moisten
a few chives

Pre-heat the oven to Gas Mark 5/190°C/375°F.
Remove the loose small fillet attached to the chicken
breast. Chop finely, and then mix with the carrot,
shallot, tarragon and yoghurt. Make an incision in
the side of the chicken breast without going all the
way through. Fill with the stuffing, then seal the
cavity with a skewer. Place the chicken in a small
ovenproof dish, and then pour the stock around it.

Cover with foil, and cook for about 20 minutes, or until the chicken is cooked.

A few minutes before the chicken is ready, cook the red onion, green pepper, turnip, carrot, celery, parsley and stock in the microwave until soft. Serve the vegetables in the centre of a plate, and then lay the chicken on them. Spoon the chicken juices over the top, and garnish with a few chives.

Chicken in Barbecue Sauce

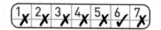

Serves 2

4 chicken thigh joints, skinned
½ medium onion, finely chopped
2 tbsp lemon juice
2 tbsp soy sauce
½ tbsp tomato purée
1 level tsp mustard powder
1 garlic clove, crushed
1 tsp low-calorie sweetener
1 tbsp low-fat yoghurt
freshly-ground black pepper (you probably won't need salt in this sauce)

Pre-heat the oven to Gas 6/200°C/400°F. Ensure the chicken joints are nice and dry, and them paint over with yoghurt and season with freshly-milled black pepper. Put them in a small, shallow roasting tin, tucking the onion in amongst them. Cook for 20-25 minutes.

Meanwhile, make up the barbecue sauce by mixing the remaining ingredients. Whisk thoroughly. Pour this over the cooked chicken, and then return to the oven. Cook for a further 15-20 minutes, basting frequently, until cooked through. Serve with a crisp, lemon-dressed salad.

Poached Chicken on a Bed of Three Kinds of Mushroom

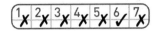

Serves 2

2x8oz (225g) chicken breasts (skin removed)
5fl oz (150ml) vegetable stock
2 shallots, chopped
1 garlic clove, finely chopped
4oz (110g) chestnut mushrooms, sliced
4oz (110g) oyster mushrooms, sliced
½ oz dried mushrooms, whichever variety you like
1 tbsp parsley, chopped
1 tsp lemon juice
salt and pepper

Soak the dried mushrooms according to the instructions on the packet. When they have finished soaking, set the mushrooms aside and add the liquid in which they were soaked to the stock. Place the stock in a shallow pan together with the chicken breasts, and poach gently until cooked.

In the meantime, cook the shallot and garlic in the microwave until soft. Transfer to a pan with a little stock to moisten if necessary, add the three mushrooms and cook until soft. Add salt, pepper, lemon juice and parsley. Slice the chicken breast on a slant. Serve on top of the mushroom mixture, and garnish with lemon slices and sprigs of parsley.

English Garden Chicken Salad

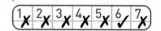

Serves 1

2x8oz (225g) chicken breasts, skin removed
½ carrot, peeled and chopped
½ onion, peeled and stuck with 3 cloves
1 stick celery, trimmed and chopped
1 level tbsp fresh tarragon, chopped
salt and freshly-ground black pepper
juice and rind of 1 lemon
an extra tbsp lemon juice
4fl oz (110ml) low-fat yoghurt
1 level tsp French mustard
1oz (25g) each of chopped radish, celery and cucumber
1 head chicory

To Garnish
lemon twists
sprigs of tarragon

Put 1 pint (570ml) water into a fairly large saucepan.
Add the carrot, onion, celery, half the tarragon, salt and
pepper, and bring to the boil. Immerse the chicken into
the liquid. Cover the pan, and then simmer until the
chicken is tender. Allow the chicken to cool in the
liquid, then remove it and set aside. Strain 10fl oz
(275ml) of the stock into a pan, add the juice of one
lemon and boil vigorously to reduce to about 3fl oz
(75ml). Leave to cool.

Meanwhile, neatly dice the chicken, put in a bowl with a combination of yoghurt, lemon juice and lemon rind and mustard. Fold gently together, then gradually stir in the cold, reduced stock. The sauce is quite thin at this point, but it should thicken with chilling. Add radish, celery and cucumber along with the remaining tarragon, then season. Chill in the fridge for at least 30 minutes before serving.

Line two individual bowls with chicory leaves, then pile the chicken salad in the centre, and garnish with the lemon twists and tarragon sprigs. Served chilled.

Chicken Curry

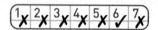

Serves 2

1 medium onion, sliced
8oz (225g) chicken breast, skin removed
2oz (50g) courgettes, sliced
2oz (50g) cauliflower florets
2oz (50g) aubergines, cut into cubes
1oz (25g) carrots, sliced
1 tbsp curry powder
5fl oz (150ml) vegetable stock
¼ tsp salt
¼ tsp low-calorie sweetener
½ tbsp tomato purée

To serve
12oz (350g) broccoli
½ tsp ground coriander
½ tsp ground cumin
salt and freshly-ground black pepper

Cook the courgettes, cauliflower, aubergines and
carrots in the microwave until slightly soft. Place in a
large saucepan, add the chicken and the curry
powder, plus a couple of tablespoons of stock if
moisture is needed, and cook for about a minute. Add
the salt, sweetener and tomato purée, and then blend
in the stock. Bring to the boil and simmer, uncovered,

for about 20 minutes, or until the chicken and vegetables are cooked.

In the meantime, cook the broccoli in the microwave, then chop it up and mix in the coriander, cumin, salt and pepper. Serve alongside the curry.

Chicken Broth

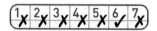

This is a really comforting winter warmer.

Serves 2

1x8oz (225g) breast of chicken
8oz (225g) in total of carrots, cauliflower florets, celery, green beans, red pepper
1 pint (570ml) vegetable stock
a bay leaf
salt and pepper
1 tbsp parsley, chopped

Chop the chicken into bite-sized pieces. Dice the vegetables. Place in a saucepan, add the stock, bay leaf and seasoning, bring to the boil, and simmer for about half-an-hour until the vegetables are soft. Sprinkle with parsley, and serve piping hot!

Russian Chicken Kebabs

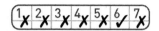

Serves 1

1x8oz (225g) breast of chicken, skin removed
6 baby beetroot
6 cherry tomatoes
1 red onion, cut into quarters lengthways
½ red pepper, cut into 6 pieces
2 bay leaves
2 kebab skewers

Boil the baby beetroots until the skins come off easily. Be sure not to pierce the skins beforehand or they will bleed. Chop the chicken into bite-sized pieces. On to each kebab skewer, thread half the chicken pieces, 3 baby beetroots, 2 bay leaves, 3 cherry tomatoes, 3 pieces of red pepper and half the onion, alternating each ingredient along the skewer. Grill until the vegetables are nicely charred and the chicken cooked through.

Mediterranean Chicken Kebabs

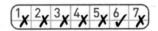

Serves 1

1x8oz (225g) breast of chicken, skin removed
1 small courgette
6 cherry tomatoes
3 shallots, cut in half
½ yellow pepper, cut into 6 pieces
½ red pepper, cut into 6 pieces
2 kebab skewers

Chop the chicken into bite-sized pieces. On to each kebab skewer, thread half the chicken pieces, 3 cherry tomatoes, 3 halves of shallot, 3 pieces of yellow pepper, 3 pieces of red pepper and half the onion, alternating each ingredient along the skewer. Grill until the vegetables are nicely charred and the chicken is cooked through. Serve with a Gazpacho Salad (page 82) on a bed of lettuce.

Fish
Dishes

Fish Dishes

Days 5 and 6 are great because you can eat as much fish as you want. You should try and avoid the really fatty kinds of fish, such as mackerel, swordfish and salmon – white-fleshed fish is the best choice. Tuna is fine, but if you want to eat tinned tuna, you can't do so in unlimited quantities. One small tin of tuna in salt water (not olive oil) is your limit.

Grilled Trout with Baked Tomatoes

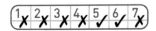

Serves 1

1 trout
3 slices of lemon
juice of 1 lemon
2 tomatoes

Pre-heat the oven to Gas Mark 5/190°C/375°F. Put the tomatoes in an oven-proof dish and cook for about 15 minutes or until cooked. Meanwhile, clean the trout well, removing the scales, gills, and the head if you wish. Put the lemon slices inside the fish and pour over the lemon juice. Grill carefully on both sides until cooked and nicely browned. Discard the lemon slices. Serve with the baked tomatoes, and the juices from the fish.

Halibut and Tomato Kebabs

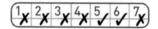

Serves 1

8oz (225g) halibut
6 cherry tomatoes
4 bay leaves
2 kebab skewers

Cut the halibut into bite-sized pieces. Thread the fish, tomatoes and bay leaves on to the skewers, alternating each ingredient along the skewer. Grill until the tomatoes are soft and the fish cooked through. What could be easier?

Tuna Medley

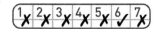

Serves 1

1 small tin tuna, preserved in salt water, *not* olive oil
½ red pepper
½ green pepper
½ orange pepper
4 radishes
4 closed-cup mushrooms
a 2-inch piece of cucumber
½ stick celery
1 tbsp low-fat dressing
a few chopped herbs
lettuce leaves, watercress and spinach

Drain the tuna well. Mix together the tuna, peppers, radishes, mushrooms, cucumber, celery and dressing. Serve the mixture on a bed of salad, watercress and spinach. Sprinkle with chopped herbs.

Sole Roulade

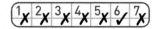

Serves 2

4 small fillets dover or lemon sole
1 tbsp chopped dill
salt and freshly-ground black pepper
5fl oz (150ml) fish stock
8oz (225g) fresh or frozen spinach (weight when cooked)
a little grated nutmeg
cauliflower florets
carrot batons
4 sprigs chervil

Pre-heat the oven to Gas Mark 4/180°C/350°F. Skin the
fillets of sole. Sprinkle the skin side of each fillet with
the dill, then roll them up from head to tail, skin side
in. Place in an oven-proof dish with the join at the
bottom so that they stay rolled up. Add the stock and
then season with pepper. Cover the dish with a lid or
foil and bake for 15 minutes. Whilst the fish is
cooking, cook and purée the spinach (if fresh) or
microwave the frozen spinach. Steam the cauliflower
florets and cook the carrots in the microwave. Drain
off any excess moisture from the spinach and season
with salt, pepper and a little grated nutmeg.

Divide the spinach into two, place a portion in the middle of each plate and place two sole roulades on top of each portion of spinach. Serve with the cauliflower and carrots, and garnish with sprigs of chervil.

Cod Steak on a Bed of Vegetable Purée

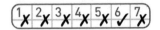

Serves 1

1x6oz (175g) cod steak
3fl oz (75ml) fish stock
2fl oz (55ml) skimmed milk
1 bay leaf
½ courgette, sliced
½ large carrot, sliced
broccoli

Pre-heat the oven to Gas Mark 4/180°C/350°F. Cook the courgette in a little vegetable stock, and in a separate pan do the same with the carrot. Place the cod in an oven-proof dish with the fish stock, skimmed milk and bay leaf. Cover and poach in the oven for 5 minutes until cooked. Whilst the fish is cooking, liquidise the carrot and courgette separately. Place the purées on a plate and lay the fish on top. Serve with some steamed broccoli.

Fresh Tuna Kebabs

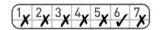

Serves 1

1 small tuna steak
4 cherry tomatoes
1 courgette
½ red pepper
½ yellow pepper
rind and juice of ½ a lemon
2 kebab skewers

Chop the tuna into 6 pieces. Place in a dish and pour the lemon juice and rind over. Chill for about an hour. Thread the fish, tomatoes and peppers on to the skewers, alternating each ingredient along the skewer. Grill until the fish is just cooked through and the vegetables nicely charred. Serve with a Cucumber and Dill Salad (page 81).

Baked Fish Italiano

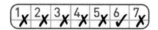

Serves 2

2 thick pieces white fish
½ medium onion, finely chopped
1 small clove garlic, crushed
7oz (200g) tin Italian tomatoes
½ tsp dried basil
2oz (50g) mushrooms, thinly sliced
juice of ½ lemon
salt and pepper
fresh basil leaves

Pre-heat the oven to Gas Mark 4/180°C/350°F. Cook the
onion and garlic, covered, in the microwave until soft. Put
the tomatoes in a pan, add the onion and garlic mixture,
season with salt and pepper and stir in the dried basil.
Bring to simmering point and cook gently for 10 minutes,
stirring occasionally. Next, stir in the sliced mushrooms
and simmer for 5-6 minutes until the mixture looks like a
thick purée.

Place the fish into a shallow baking dish, season with
salt and pepper, and sprinkle a little lemon juice on each
piece. Spoon an equal quantity of the tomato mixture on to
each piece of fish. Cover the dish with foil and bake for
about 15 minutes – the precise length of cooking will
depend on the thickness of the fish. Transfer to a plate and
garnish with fresh basil, and serve with a fresh herb salad.

Haddock with Leeks

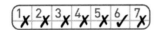

Serves 2

12oz (350g) haddock
1 dsp lemon juice
salt and pepper
2 small leeks
3oz (75g) mushrooms
3oz (75g) Chinese cabbage
about 7 tbsp water or vegetable stock

Cut the fish into 2 pieces, sprinkle with the lemon juice and then season. Finely chop the leeks, mushrooms and cabbage. Place 4 tbsp water or vegetable stock in a saucepan, add the leeks, cover, and cook over a gentle heat for 8 minutes, stirring occasionally. Add the mushrooms and cabbage, cover again, and cook gently for 5 minutes. Season to taste. Place the fish on top of the vegetables in the pan. Add another 3 tbsp water or stock, cover and cook for about 5 minutes until the fish is cooked through. Lift out the fish portions and arrange them on 2 plates, surrounded by the vegetables.

Oriental Grilled Fish

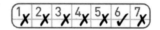

Serves 1

1 trout
1 tbsp soy sauce
1 tbsp lime or lemon juice
8fl oz (220ml) water
2 spring onions, cut in diagonal chunks
1 garlic clove, peeled and finely chopped
1 inch piece ginger, sliced thinly
1 small red pepper, de-seeded and sliced
1 green pepper, de-seeded and sliced
4oz (110g) oyster or large button mushrooms, sliced
1 tbsp ground turmeric
a little vegetable stock
fresh coriander or parsley to garnish

Blend the soy sauce, lime juice and water together. Cook the onion, garlic and ginger in the microwave. Toss the peppers and mushrooms in a little vegetable stock until cooked but still slightly crisp. Drain the peppers and mushrooms, and add to the onions, garlic and ginger in a pan. Add the turmeric and cook for about a minute. Add the soy sauce mixture and season to taste. Keep warm.

Wash and dry the fish, and place under a pre-heated grill. Grill for about 5 minutes on each side, turning carefully. Spoon the sauce over the grilled fish and serve garnished with the fresh herbs.

Haddock en Papillotte

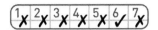

Serves 2

2x4oz (110g) haddock steaks
1 carrot, peeled and cut into julienne strips
1 leek, cut into thin strips
a few slices of fresh ginger
1 tbsp soy sauce
½ garlic clove, crushed
½ tsp Worcestershire sauce
2 tsp lemon juice
freshly-ground black pepper
1 tbsp chopped parsley

Pre-heat the oven to Gas 4/180°C/350°F. Cut two pieces of greaseproof paper or foil, large enough to enclose the steaks. Place one steak on top of each, and cover with the vegetables and ginger. Mix together the soy sauce, garlic, Worcestershire sauce and lemon juice, pour over the fish and season well with pepper. Fold the paper or foil around the fish, and scrunch up at the top to seal well. Place on a baking tray. Bake for 15 minutes. Unwrap the fish, sprinkle with parsley and serve.

Hot
Vegetable
Dishes

Hot Vegetable Dishes

One of the best things about the Cabbage Soup Diet is that you can, on certain days, eat unlimited quantities of fresh vegetables. Here are 10 new and interesting ways of cooking them.

Green Bean and Savoury Salad

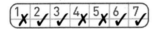

The herb savoury can be found in two different varieties – summer savoury (an annual) and winter savoury (a perennial). It is a herb traditionally used in conjunction with beans, and may often be used to replace sage.

Serves 1

8oz (225g) green beans
5fl oz (150ml) vegetable stock
2 tsp savoury, chopped
1 dsp low-fat yoghurt
freshly-ground black pepper

Combine the savoury and the yoghurt. Cook the beans in the vegetable stock, drain and transfer to a warm plate. Season well with black pepper, and top with the yoghurt and savoury. Serve immediately.

Beetroot with Rosemary

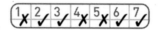

Serves 4

3 medium beetroot, peeled and quartered
6 medium red onions, peeled and quartered
4 large sprigs rosemary
15fl oz (450ml) vegetable stock
2 tbsp raspberry vinegar
salt and freshly-ground black pepper
1 tbsp low-fat natural yoghurt
rosemary sprigs to garnish

Partially cook the onions in the microwave with the
rosemary, covered. Put the stock and vinegar in a pan,
add the beetroot and onions with the rosemary. Bring
to the boil and simmer for one hour until the beetroot
is tender. Remove the lid and boil steadily until the
liquid reduces to a glaze. Season and discard the
rosemary. Transfer to a warm serving dish, spoon the
yoghurt over, and garnish with rosemary sprigs.

Carrots and Artichoke Hearts

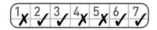

This would be particularly good served with one of the chicken dishes on Day 6.

Serves 1

2 carrots, peeled, sliced and cooked in a little vegetable stock
2 artichoke hearts, heated
2 tsp lemon juice
salt and pepper
2 tbsp low-fat natural yoghurt
1 dsp chives, chopped

Purée the artichoke hearts and carrots along with the vegetable stock together in a liquidiser. Mix in the lemon juice and yoghurt, and season with salt and pepper. Garnish with the chopped chives.

Oriental Vegetables

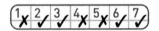

Serves 2

1 large carrot, peeled and cut into batons
1 courgette, peeled and cut into batons
2 sticks celery, trimmed and cut into batons
1 leek, cut into ½-inch pieces
a small piece of ginger, peeled and sliced
2 tbsp soy sauce
1 tsp five spice powder
juice and grated rind of ½ lime
salt and pepper
1 dsp fresh coriander, chopped

Cook the vegetables in the microwave until they are cooked through, but retain some bite. In the meantime, mix the ginger and spices into the soy sauce. Add the rind and juice of the lime. Pour over the hot vegetables and toss. Garnish with chopped coriander.

Spicy Garden Vegetables

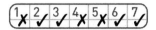

Serves 2

4oz (110g) broccoli pieces
4oz (110g) cauliflower florets
4oz (110g) brussels sprouts
5fl oz (150ml) low-fat natural yoghurt
½ tsp ground cumin
½ tsp ground coriander
1 dsp fresh coriander, chopped

Steam the vegetables until cooked *al dente*. Mix the spices with the yoghurt, and pour over the vegetables. Garnish with chopped coriander.

Stuffed Peppers

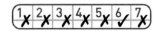

Serves 2

1 red pepper
1 yellow pepper
8 cherry tomatoes
1 large garlic clove
2 small mushrooms
4 sprigs fresh basil

Pre-heat the oven to Gas 4/180°C/350°F. Cut the peppers in half lengthways, removing the seeds. Chop 2 sprigs of the basil. Chop the mushrooms. Slice the garlic finely. Divide the garlic, mushrooms, basil and tomatoes between the peppers. Bake for 20 minutes. Serve garnished with the remaining basil sprigs.

Asparagus with Yoghurt and Lemon Dressing

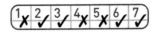

Serves 1

6 asparagus stalks
5fl oz (150ml) yoghurt
rind and juice of ½ lemon

Gently scrape the asparagus stalks. Place in a pan of cold water, bring to the boil, and boil for 1 minute. Remove the asparagus and plunge into iced water. When ready to serve, bring the hot water back up to the boil, add the asparagus and boil for about another minute until tender. Mix the lemon juice with the yoghurt, and serve with the asparagus, sprinkled with the zest of the lemon.

Tomatoes Farcis

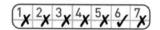

Serves 1

2 large tomatoes
2 shallots
2oz (50g) button mushrooms
1 tsp fresh herbs, chopped
2 tsp tomato ketchup
1 tbsp lemon juice
a few chopped chives

Pre-heat the oven to Gas Mark 4/180°C/350°F. Chop the shallots and mushrooms finely, and cook gently in a little lemon juice. Add the chopped herbs and the ketchup. Cut the tops off the tomatoes and spoon out the seeds and juice. Fill the hollow tomatoes with the mixture and bake for 15-20 minutes. Serve garnished with chopped chives.

Baked Onions

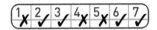

Serves 1

1 large onion, peeled
1oz (25g) chestnut mushrooms
½ garlic clove
1 dsp fresh parsley, chopped
1 tsp tomato ketchup
a few drops of Tabasco sauce
3fl oz (75ml) vegetable stock

Pre-heat the oven to Gas Mark 4/180°C/350°F. Remove
the end of each onion and then push out the centre
from the onion. You will be left with the empty shell
of the onion. Chop the onion that you have removed,
and mix with all the other ingredients. Spoon the
mixture into the cavity of the onion. There will be a
little mixture left over. Place the onion in a small
oven-proof dish, and surround with the stock and the
excess filling. Bake for about 20 minutes until tender,
keeping an eye on the liquid – if it looks like drying
out, add a little more. Serve the onion with the juices
poured over it.

Hot Vegetable Salad

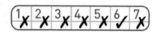

Serves 1

1 leek
2 spring onions
2 medium tomatoes
½ red pepper
½ yellow pepper
5fl oz (150ml) vegetable stock
1 tbsp fresh parsley, chopped

Pre-heat the oven to Gas Mark 4/180°C/350°F. Cut the leeks and the spring onions on the slant about ½ inch long. Cut the tomatoes in half, and the peppers in strips. Put in an oven-proof dish with the stock, cover and cook for about 30 minutes. Serve sprinkled with the parsley.

Cold
Vegetable
Dishes

Cold Vegetable Dishes

Salads play an important part in the Cabbage Soup Diet. You'll be eating a lot of them on your vegetable days, so let's make them tasty!

Cucumber and Dill Salad

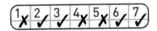

This is a very refreshing salad which can be made in advance and kept in the fridge.

Serves 1

½ large cucumber
salt
2 tbsp white wine vinegar
sweetener to taste
1 tbsp fresh dill, chopped
dill sprigs to garnish

Peel the cucumber, and slice as thinly as possible. Place in a colander, sprinkling each layer with salt. Cover with a plate, and place a weight on top. Leave to stand for 30 minutes to remove excess water. Put the vinegar and sweetener in a saucepan with 2 tbsp water. Bring to the boil for 1 minute and then leave to cool. Rinse the salted cucumber with cold water. Pat dry, and put in a serving dish. Stir the dill into the dressing, pour over the cucumber and mix well. Cover the bowl and leave in the fridge to marinate for at least two hours. When serving, garnish with the fresh dill sprigs.

Gazpacho Salad

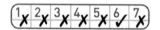

Serves 4

8oz (225g) ripe tomatoes, skinned
½ large green pepper
½ large yellow pepper
¼ small cucumber
a few radishes, cut into quarters
2 small garlic cloves
3 tbsp tomato juice
1 tbsp red wine vinegar
a good pinch cayenne pepper or chilli powder
salt and freshly-ground black pepper

Core and dice the peeled tomatoes into ½ inch cubes. De-seed the peppers and cut them into thin strips. Cut the cucumber into strips of the same size. Make the dressing by combining the garlic, tomato juice, vinegar, cayenne pepper or chilli powder, salt and pepper. Arrange the vegetables on a serving dish, pour over a small amount of the dressing, then chill for 30 minutes. Remove the chilled salad from the fridge and pour the remaining dressing over it. Garnish with the radishes.

Belgian Salad

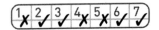

Serves 2

3 sticks celery, chopped
4 spring onions, chopped
6 brussels sprouts, chopped
2 carrots, grated
1 tbsp low-fat dressing, to which a little lemon juice may be added
2 tsp chives, chopped
salt and freshly-ground black pepper

Combine the celery, onions, sprouts and carrots. Pour over the dressing, season, and garnish with the chives.

Salade aux Fines Herbes

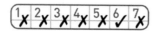

Serves 1

2 medium tomatoes, sliced
3-inch piece cucumber, sliced
½ orange pepper, sliced
½ yellow pepper, sliced
1 tbsp fresh mixed herbs, chopped
2 tbsp lemon juice
2 tbsp water
a little sweetener
½ bunch watercress
sprig of basil

Arrange the watercress on a plate. Arrange the tomatoes, cucumber and peppers attractively on the watercress. Combine the herbs with the lemon juice, water and sweetener, pour over the salad and garnish with a sprig of basil.

Green Asparagus Salad

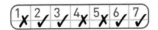

Serves 1

6 stalks asparagus
1 courgette
2 tbsp vegetable stock
1 tbsp lemon juice
salt and freshly-ground black pepper
lamb's lettuce

Gently scrape the stems of the asparagus. Place them in a pan of cold water, bring to the boil, and boil for 1 minute. Remove the asparagus, keeping the water in the pan, and plunge immediately into iced water. Bring the pan of hot water back up to the boil, and boil the asparagus for a further minute. Remove, and allow to cool. This process of blanching and refreshing the asparagus will keep it nice and green.

Peel and slice the courgette, and cook gently in the stock. Liquidise, adding lemon juice to taste, salt and pepper. Leave to cool. Place the courgette purée in the middle of a plate, top with the cold asparagus, and surround with lamb's lettuce.

Popeye's Salad

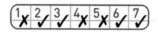

This is called Popeye's Salad because of the nutritious inclusion of raw baby spinach. Whether Popeye himself would like it is a different matter – olive oil is strictly forbidden!

Serves 1

3 handfuls baby spinach, stalks removed
1 small punnet cress
6 radishes, sliced
¼ cucumber
2 tsp lemon juice
½ tsp French mustard
a little vegetable stock, if needed

Wash the spinach and cress, dry carefully and mix together on a large plate. Peel the cucumber and then liquidise with the lemon juice and mustard. If too thick, add a little vegetable stock. Pour over the salad, and garnish with the radishes.

Artichoke Hearts with Herb Dressing

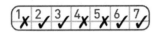

Serves 1

1 tin artichoke hearts in water (you will need about 4 hearts in all)
juice of ½ lemon
a little stock
1 tbsp fresh mixed herbs, chopped

Place 3 of the artichoke hearts on a plate and sprinkle with a little lemon juice. Liquidise the remaining heart with the rest of the lemon juice and enough stock to make a pouring consistency. Add the chopped herbs and pour over the artichoke hearts.

Crudités with a Trio of Dips

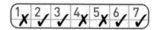

Serve these three dips with your choice of raw free vegetables – some suggestions are made here.

For the Crudités
small sprigs raw cauliflower
batons of raw carrot
batons of raw courgette
batons of celery
baby mushrooms

For the Spicy Courgette Dip
1 courgette
2 tbsp vegetable stock
¼ tsp cumin
¼ tsp coriander
pinch of cayenne pepper
salt and freshly-ground black pepper

Peel and slice the courgette. Cook gently in the stock. Liquidise, adding the spices, then season to taste.

For the Raita
2oz (50g) peeled cucumber
1 spring onion, chopped
1 small garlic clove, crushed
5fl oz (150ml) low-fat natural yoghurt

a good pinch of cayenne pepper
a pinch of cumin seeds
salt and freshly-ground black pepper

Cut the cucumber lengthways, then slice thinly.
Sprinkle with salt and leave for an hour by which time
a lot of liquid will have been expelled. Drain, and dry
with kitchen paper. Combine the cucumber, spring
onion, garlic and yoghurt. Season with salt and
pepper, transfer to a serving bowl and sprinkle the
spices on top. Cover and chill before serving.

For the Christmas Dip
1 carrot, sliced and cooked in 2 tbsp vegetable stock
2 tsp lemon juice
½ tsp cinnamon
½ tsp mixed spice
zest of ½ an orange

Liquidise all the ingredients together. Add a little stock,
if necessary, to make a good consistency.

Russian Salad

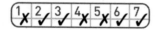

Serves 1 as a main course

1 large beetroot
1 medium red onion
2 tbsp red wine vinegar
a little sweetener
4fl oz (110ml) low-fat natural yoghurt
1 tsp chopped chives

Boil the beetroot, making sure not to pierce the skin.
Cook until the skin can be removed easily. Put into
cold water, remove the skin, and allow to cool. Peel
and slice the red onion, put into a pan of cold water
and bring to the boil. Boil for 1 minute and drain. Mix
the vinegar with a little sweetener. Slice the cold
beetroot. Sprinkle both the beetroot and the red onion
with the sweetened vinegar. Arrange the beetroot in a
circle around the serving plate, put the red onion in
the middle, top with the yoghurt, and sprinkle with
the chives.

Welsh Salad

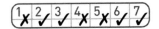

Serves 1

8 young, thin leeks
black pepper
1 tbsp low-calorie dressing

Blanch the leeks in boiling salted water for 5-6
minutes. Drain carefully, chill well, sprinkle with
freshly-ground black pepper, and dress with the low-
calorie dressing.

Hot Fruit Dishes

Hot Fruit Dishes

A lot of people forget that fruit is quite delicious when baked, grilled or poached. The recipes in this section offer some brilliant ways of spicing up your fruit days. A lot of them can be eaten at any time of the day, and they make particularly hearty breakfasts.

Baked Apple

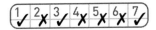

This is everyone's favourite – the cinnamon makes it particularly moreish!

Serves 1

1 large apple
½ tsp cinnamon
1 tsp sweetener
1 dsp blueberries

Pre-heat the oven to Gas Mark 4/180°C/350°F. Core the apple. Put in an oven-proof dish with a little water or pure, unsweetened apple juice. Mix the berries, sweetener and cinnamon together, and stuff the cavity of the apple. Bake until soft but keeping its shape. This can also be cooked in the microwave according to the manufacturer's instructions.

Baked Banana

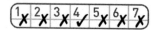

This is one of the most delicious things you can eat! Try it once and you'll be coming back for more, diet or no diet. It's also a particularly good way of using up bananas that are past their best.

Serves 1

1 banana

Pre-heat the oven to Gas Mark 4/180°C/350°F. Place the banana on a baking tray and bake for 15 minutes or until soft. The skin will go black. When cooked, remove from the oven, make an incision along the length of the banana and eat from the skin with a teaspoon.

Two of a Kind Pudding

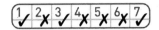

Serves 2

2 peaches, halved and stoned
2 nectarines, halved and stoned
5fl oz (150ml) orange juice
½ vanilla pod
a few sprigs of mint

Heat the orange juice with the vanilla pod. Add fruit,
cover, and poach gently on the hob until the fruit is
soft when pierced. Serve with the poaching juice
poured over and garnish with mint.

Grilled Grapefruit

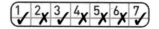

Serves 1

½ prepared grapefruit
¼ tsp cinnamon
¼ tsp ground ginger
a sprig of mint (ginger mint is particularly recommended)

Place the grapefruit under a medium grill until it
begins to bubble and go brown. Sprinkle with the
cinnamon and ginger, garnish with the mint, and
serve.

Grilled Orangey Apricots

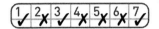

Serves 1

2-3 apricots
3fl oz (75ml) fresh orange juice

Halve the apricots and remove the stones. Place under a medium grill until nicely caramelised. In the meantime, heat the orange juice. Serve the apricots with the juice poured over, and sprinkled with a little sweetener if desired.

Grilled Pineapple

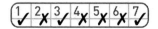

Serves 1

½ a fresh pineapple, skinned, sliced and cored
2 tsp fresh mint, chopped
2fl oz (55ml) orange juice

Grill the pineapple under a medium grill until nicely caramelised. Heat the orange juice, and serve the pineapple with the juice poured over and sprinkled with fresh mint.

Hot Ruby Salad

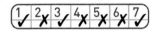

Serves 2-4

4oz (110g) strawberries
4oz (110g) cherries
4oz (110g) plums
2oz (55g) seedless red grapes
2 tbsp orange juice

Pre-heat the oven to Gas Mark 4/180°C/350°F. If the strawberries are large, halve them. Halve and stone the plums. Place all the ingredients in an ovenproof dish and cook until the juices start to run.

Citrus Warmer

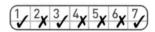

This makes an excellent breakfast on a cold winter's day.

Serves 1

1 orange, peeled and segmented
1 pink grapefruit, peeled and segmented
1 tangerine, peeled and segmented

Pre-heat the oven to Gas Mark 4/180°C/350°F. Cut away the skin and pith from the orange and grapefruit, and place in an oven-proof dish with the tangerine segments. Bake in the oven for about 10 minutes, and serve piping hot.

Tangerine Dream

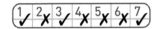

Serves 2-4

1 apple, peeled, cored and sliced
1 tbsp blueberries
2 nectarines, sliced
2 peaches, sliced
6 strawberries, halved
1 tangerine, peeled and segmented
6 cherries
juice of 2 tangerines
1 dsp lemon thyme, chopped

Place all the ingredients in a saucepan, cover and poach gently until the fruit is softened and the juices start to run. Serve with the lemon thyme sprinkled over.

Pineapple and Apple

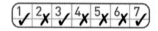

Serves 1

1 slice prepared pineapple
1 apple
juice of ½ orange
a sprig of mint (pineapple mint is particularly delicious)

Peel, core and slice the apple. Poach gently in the orange juice until soft. Purée with the orange juice and keep warm. Grill the pineapple slice and serve on top of the apple puree. Garnish with a sprig of mint.

Cold Fruit Dishes

Cold Fruit Dishes

Don't get stuck in the rut of unimaginative fruit salads on your fruit days. This section does contain a recipe for a Classic Fruit Salad, but there is also a selection of other interesting cold fruit dishes, all of them really easy.

Chinese Gooseberry Salad

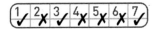

Most people know the Chinese Gooseberry as kiwi fruit. It comes orginally from China, but is now, of course, mainly cultivated in New Zealand. Peel before serving.

Serves 1-2

½ small pineapple, cut into cubes
1 mandarin, broken into segments
6 strawberries
1 kiwi fruit
juice of ½ orange

Cut up the fruit, arrange in a bowl, and pour over the orange juice.

Florida Cocktail

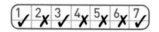

Serves 1

1 orange
½ grapefruit
1 tbsp low-fat dressing
1 tsp mint, finely chopped

Peel and segment the fruit, removing all the pith.
Arrange alternate segments in a bowl. Mix the mint
with the dressing, and pour over.

Melon and Ginger

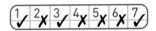

Melon and Ginger is a classic combination.

Serves 1

½ small melon
½ tsp powdered ginger
2 tbsp orange juice

Remove the seeds from the melon. Mix the orange juice and ginger together, and pour into the cavity. Serve at room temperature.

Pineapple and Strawberry Surprise

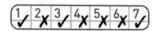

Serves 1

2 slices fresh pineapple
½ small punnet strawberries
mint to garnish (try pineapple mint – it's delicious)

Purée 1 slice of the pineapple and put into a dish.
Place the other slice on it. Purée all but one
strawberry. Pour over the pineapple. Garnish with
mint and the reserved strawberry.

Banana Whip

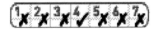

This is a great way of using up your banana allowance on day 4.

Serves 1

2 bananas
4fl oz (110ml) low-fat natural yoghurt
½ vanilla pod

Remove the seeds from the vanilla pod. Mash the seeds well with the bananas, and fold into the yoghurt. Could there be an easier recipe?

Salad of Berries

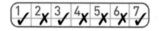

Serves 1

2oz (50g) strawberries
1oz (25g) raspberries
1oz (25g) blackberries
1oz (25g) blueberries
a sprig of basil

Purée the strawberries, reserving one. Arrange the berries over the purée. Garnish with a sprig of basil and the reserved strawberry.

Fresh Fruit Yoghurt

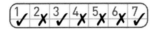

You could do any combination of this – but here is a particularly good and simple one!

Serves 1

2oz (50g) strawberries
2oz (50g) raspberries
8fl oz (220ml) low-fat natural yoghurt

Purée the strawberries and raspberries together. Mix with the yoghurt and serve.

Apple and Blackberry Pie

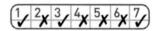

Serves 1

1 large eating apple
2oz (50g) dessert blackberries
a little lemon juice

Peel and core the apple. Cut in half. Slice one half of apple, and sprinkle with a little lemon juice to stop it going brown. Stew the other half of the apple in a little water until it is soft, and then purée. Put the puréed apple in a ramekin, and then layer the blackberries on top. Cover with the sliced apple, and put under a medium grill, until the apple is nicely caramelised. Allow to cool, and then serve.

TIP: This is equally delicious served hot!

Cantaloupe Island

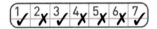

Serves 1

½ cantaloupe melon
2oz (50g) cherries, stoned
2oz (50g) seedless green grapes
1 tbsp orange juice

Remove the seeds from the melon. Fill the cavity with
the cherries and grapes. Sprinkle with the orange juice
and serve.

Classic Fruit Salad

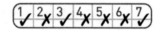

Serves 1-2

1 slice honeydew melon, cut into chunks
1 nectarine
½ tangerine, segmented
½ apple, cored and chopped
8 strawberries, sliced
6 seedless green grapes
juice of one orange
1 dsp fresh mint, chopped

Combine the melon, nectarine, tangerine, apple, strawberries and grapes in a serving bowl. Mix the orange juice and mint, and pour over the fruit before serving.

Fruit and Vegetable Combinations

Fruit and Vegetable Combinations

These dishes are designed for days 3 and 7, when you can have unlimited quantities of free fruit and free vegetables.

Melon, Cucumber and Grape Salad

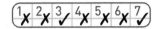

Serves 2

½ cucumber
½ canteloupe melon
½ Charentais melon
1 slice red watermelon
2oz (50g) black seedless grapes
2oz (50g) green seedless grapes
1 tbsp fresh mint, chopped
1 tbsp balsamic vinegar
3 tbsp orange juice
salt and freshly-ground black pepper
sprigs of basil to garnish

Peel the cucumber and cut in half lengthways. Scoop
out the seeds and cut into slices about ¼-inch thick.
Place in a colander and sprinkle with a little salt.
Leave for about 20 minutes to drain some of the
juices. Thoroughly rinse and dry.

Remove the seeds from the melons and, using a
melon scoop, make into balls. Combine the cucumber,
melon balls, grapes and mint in a bowl. Mix together
the vinegar and orange juice, season with salt and
pepper, and use to dress the salad. Toss and serve,
garnished with a sprig of basil.

Winter Salad

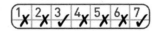

Serves 1-2

4oz (110g) young brussels sprouts
4oz (110g) white of leek
3 apricots
1 Cox's apple, quartered and cored
juice and zest of ½ lemon
1 tbsp fresh parsley, chopped
1 tbsp low-fat dressing
2 tbsp orange juice
salt and freshly-ground black pepper

Shred the sprouts finely and place in a large salad bowl. Slice the leeks finely, separating them into rings, and place in the bowl. Slice the apples, coat them with lemon juice, and add to the bowl. Halve and stone the apricots, chop into small pieces and add to the bowl. Add the parsley and seasoning. Combine the dressing, orange juice and lemon zest, and add to the salad. Toss and serve.

Layered Peach, Cucumber & Pepper Salad

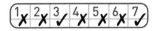

Serves 2

½ oak leaf lettuce
2 ripe peaches, halved, stoned and thinly sliced
a 2-inch piece cucumber, thinly sliced
½ red pepper, de-seeded and thinly sliced
3oz (75g) mushroom caps, cleaned and thinly sliced
3oz (75g) carrot, peeled and finely grated
12 black seedless grapes
1 dsp fresh herbs, chopped

For the Peach Dressing
1 ripe peach
1 tsp prepared English mustard
1½ tbsp white wine vinegar

First make the dressing. Gently poach the peach in a little water until soft. Liquidise with the mustard and vinegar. Heat, and keep warm. Meanwhile, place the salad ingredients in layers in a salad bowl, with the lettuce leaves on the bottom. Pour the warm dressing over, and garnish with the fresh herbs.

Braised Celery with Orange

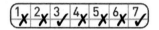

Serves 2

1 heart of celery, trimmed, cleaned and cut in half
segments cut from 1 large orange, rind and pith removed
juice of ½ orange
2oz (50g) vegetable stock
1 tsp fresh rosemary, chopped

Place the prepared celery in a suitable microwave
dish, together with the orange segments, orange juice
and stock. Cook until tender. Sprinkle with the
rosemary before serving.

Beetroot and Orange Salad

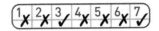

Serves 1-2

8oz (225g) beetroot
1 large orange
1 tsp celery seeds
2 tbsp white wine vinegar
2½fl oz (75ml) water
a little sweetener
juice of ½ orange
salt and freshly-ground black pepper

Boil the beetroot until the skins can be easily removed,
taking care not to puncture the skin at any stage. Peel and
set aside to cool.

To make the dressing, lightly crush the celery seeds in
a mortar and place them in a saucepan. Add the vinegar,
water, orange juice and sweetener. Boil until the liquid has
reduced to about 2 tablespoons. Strain, and set aside to
cool.

With a zester, remove long strips of zest from the
orange and set aside. Using a sharp knife, peel the orange,
cutting away the pith and the skin. Slice the orange into
rings, catching any juices in a bowl to add to the dressing.

Thinly slice the beetroot, cubing a small amount to set
in the centre of the dish. Arrange the orange and beetroot
slices alternately around the dish. Place the cubed
beetroot in the middle, pour over the dressing, and garnish
with the orange zest.

Marinated Mushroom, Apricot and Artichoke Salad

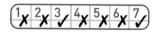

Serves 1

4 tinned artichoke hearts
8oz (225g) button mushrooms
2 tbsp lemon juice
1 tsp coriander seeds
¼ tsp cumin seeds
1 garlic clove
1 tbsp cider vinegar
1 apricot, poached in a little water until tender
a little vegetable stock, if needed
red and white onion rings
fresh coriander leaves, chopped

Trim the base of the mushroom stalks and wipe clean. Drain the tinned artichoke hearts and put them in a large bowl. Bring a saucepan of water to the boil, add 1 tbsp lemon juice and the mushrooms, and cook for 1 minute. Drain the mushrooms and rinse them in cold water. Pat dry and add to the artichokes.

Crush the coriander, cumin seeds and garlic in a mortar. Purée the poached apricot in a liquidiser, put in a pan with the crushed mixture and cook for 1 minute. Add the remaining lemon juice and vinegar, and cook for a further minute or two. Add a

124

little stock if needed. Stir this mixture over the mushrooms and artichoke. Cover and chill for about 4 hours. To serve, place the mixture in a salad bowl and garnish with the onion rings and coriander.

Spinach Medley

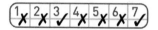

Serves 1

a handful baby spinach, stalks removed
2oz (50g) mushrooms, diced
½ red pepper, diced
½ yellow pepper, diced
8 green seedless grapes
1 tangerine
juice of ½ orange
1 tbsp low-fat dressing
salt and freshly-ground black pepper

Rinse the spinach thoroughly and pat dry with kitchen paper. Arrange the spinach on a plate. Combine the chopped mushrooms, peppers, grapes and tangerine with the orange juice and dressing. Season with salt and pepper, and arrange in the middle of the plate on top of the spinach.

Melon Salad Basket

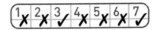

Serves 1

½ melon, seeds removed
1 stick celery, chopped
2 inches cucumber, peeled and chopped
3 radishes, chopped
1 tsp fresh mixed herbs, chopped
1 tbsp orange juice
½ tbsp lemon juice

Fill the melon with the chopped vegetables. Combine
the orange and lemon juice, pour this over the melon,
and sprinkle with the herbs.

Fruity Endive Salad

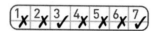

Serves 1

1 cooked beetroot
1 endive
½ pineapple
½ punnet small cress
juice of 1 orange
1 tbsp balsamic vinegar

Arrange the endive around a plate. Chop the beetroot and pineapple into dice and mix together. Place in the middle of the plate. Top with the cress. Combine the orange juice and balsamic vinegar and pour over the salad.

Crunchy Combination Salad

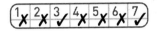

Serves 1

heart of 1 small round lettuce
3 inches cucumber, chopped
1 Cox's apple, cored and chopped
1 stick celery, chopped
1 tangerine
1 tbsp low-calorie dressing
1 tbsp orange juice
1 tsp fresh chives, chopped

Combine the dressing, orange juice and chives. Mix the lettuce, apple, celery and tangerine in a salad bowl. Add the dressing and serve.

Jacket
Potatoes

Jacket Potatoes

Everyone loves jacket potatoes, and on day 2 of the Cabbage Soup Diet you're allowed a large baked potato and unlimited free vegetables. Here are just a few ideas for serving them.

Jacket Potato with Yoghurt and Chives

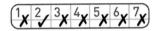

Serves 1

1 large baked potato
1 tbsp low-fat natural yoghurt
1 tsp fresh chives, chopped
salt and pepper

Combine the yoghurt and chives, season well with salt and pepper, spoon over the potato and serve immediately.

Crunchy Jacket Potato

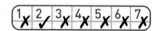

Serves 1

1 large baked potato
½ stick celery
2 spring onions
1 tbsp low-fat dressing
salt and pepper
1 tsp chives, chopped

Chop the celery and spring onions finely, mix with the dressing, season to taste, and spoon over the potato. Sprinkle with chives.

Jacket Potato with Rosemary

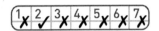

Serves 1

1 large baked potato
½ green pepper, finely chopped
4 radishes, finely chopped
1 tsp fresh rosemary, chopped
1 tbsp low-fat natural yoghurt
salt and pepper

Mix the ingredients together, season to taste, and spoon over the potato.

Spicy Potato Skins

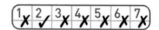

Serves 1

1 large baked potato
1 shallot, finely chopped
½ garlic clove, finely chopped
1 tbsp low-fat natural yoghurt
¼ tsp each of ground cumin, ground coriander and ground turmeric
salt and freshly-ground black pepper
1 tsp fresh coriander, chopped

Cut the baked potato in half, scoop out the flesh, and return the potato skins to the oven. Whilst they are baking, cook the shallot and garlic covered in the microwave. Mix the cooked shallot mixture with the yoghurt, spices and cooked potato. Season to taste. When the insides of the potato skins are nicely browned, fill with the mixture. Return to the oven to heat through, and serve with the chopped coriander.

Jacket Potato al Funghi

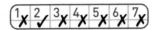

Serves 1

1 large baked potato
2oz (50g) button mushrooms, finely chopped
1 tbsp fresh parsley, finely chopped
2 tsp lemon juice
1 tbsp low-fat natural yoghurt
salt and freshly-ground black pepper

Combine all the filling ingredients, season to taste, and spoon over the baked potato.

Minty Jacket Potato

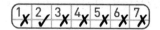

Serves 1

1 large baked potato
1 spring onion, finely chopped
2-inch piece of cucumber, peeled, de-seeded and chopped
2-inch piece of celery, finely chopped
1 tsp fresh mint, chopped
1 tbsp low-calorie dressing
salt and freshly-ground black pepper
small cress to garnish

Combine the onion, cucumber, celery, mint and dressing. Season to taste. Spoon over the baked potato and garnish with the cress.

Jacket Potato with a Vegetable Medley

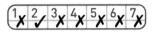

Serves 1

1 large baked potato
1 small carrot, grated
½ small courgette, finely chopped
1 small sprig cauliflower, finely chopped
¼ tsp cinnamon
1 tbsp low-fat natural yoghurt
salt and freshly-ground black pepper

Mix the cinnamon into the yoghurt, and fold in the vegetables. Season to taste. Spoon over the baked potato.

Jacket Potato with a Garden Salad

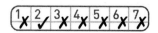

Serves 1

1 large baked potato
1 tbsp low-fat natural yoghurt
1 tsp celery leaves, chopped
1 tsp chives, chopped
a small handful of three of the following: baby spinach,
kale, endive, chard, cress, chicory, sorrel, watercress
a little lemon juice
salt and freshly-ground black pepper

Combine the yoghurt, celery leaves and chives.
Season well. Make a salad of whichever green leaves
you chose, and dress in a little lemon juice. Spoon the
yoghurt mixture over the potato, and serve with the
salad on one side.

Jacket Potato with Baked Vegetables

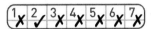

Serves 1

1 large baked potato
the white part of a small leek, sliced thinly
1 spring onion, sliced
¼ pepper, sliced
1 tbsp low-fat dressing
salt and freshly-ground black pepper

Bake the leek, onion and pepper until slightly charred. Mix with the dressing, season to taste, and spoon over the potato.

Sage and Onion Jacket Potato

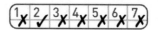

Serves 1

1 large baked potato
½ onion, chopped
½ garlic clove, chopped
2 tsp fresh sage, finely chopped
salt and freshly-ground black pepper

Cook the onion and the garlic covered in the microwave. Mix in the sage, season to taste, and spoon over the baked potato.

Drinks

Drinks

You can have as much black tea and coffee as you want on the Cabbage Soup Diet, but a lot of people have complained that it gets a bit boring. So why not create something more interesting to drink? Here are ten great ways of staving off your thirst...

Banana Milk Shake

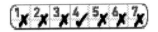

You can only have this on day 4, but it's a delicious way of getting through all those bananas and all that milk!

Serves 1

1 banana
8fl oz (220ml) skimmed milk

Blitz the banana and the milk together in a liquidiser. Pour into a cold glass and serve.

Iced Tea with Mint

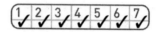

This is delicious and refreshing whether you're on a diet or not!

Serves 2-3

good tea leaves
boiling water
crushed ice
2 tsp mint leaves, crushed
thin slices of lemon or orange

Make strong tea using 1 tsp tea for each person. Infuse in boiling water and leave to stand in a warm place for 3 minutes. Strain, chill, and pour over crushed ice. Add thin slices of lemon or orange and crushed mint leaves.

Indian Yoghurt Drink

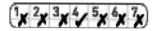

Day 4 is the only day you're allowed milk and yoghurt together, so why not treat yourself with this unusual drink?

Serves 1

8fl oz (220ml) low-fat natural yoghurt
8fl oz (220ml) skimmed milk
4 drops rosewater
½ tsp ground cardamom
½ tsp cinnamon
a little sweetener
4 ice cubes

Place all the ingredients in a liquidiser. Add 2fl oz (50ml) cold water. Liquidise, and pour into a tall glass. Serve chilled.

Tropical Fruit Punch

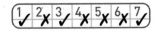

Serves 4

½ large ripe pineapple
4 large juicy oranges
4 kiwi fruit
crushed ice to serve
orange slices and pineapple leaves for garnish

Peel the pineapple (reserving a few leaves), remove the woody core, and cut into pieces. Peel and chop the kiwi fruit. Place the pineapple and kiwi fruit in a liquidiser and blend until smooth. Pass through a sieve to remove the fibres and the seeds. Cut the oranges in half and squeeze out the juice. You will need about 15fl oz (450ml). Mix the juices together. Half fill your serving glasses with crushed ice, and decorate with the orange slices and pineapple leaves.

Virgin Mary

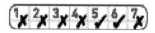

Home-made tomato juice makes an excellent aperitif.

Serves 2

6 tomatoes, chopped
2fl oz (50 ml) water
small stick of celery
½ bay leaf
2 sprigs parsley
2 sprigs basil
a pinch of salt
a pinch of paprika
a dash of Worcestershire sauce
a couple of drops of Tabasco sauce
a squeeze of lemon juice

Place the tomatoes, water, celery, bay leaf, parsley
and basil in a saucepan and simmer until the tomatoes
are nice and soft. Strain through a sieve, and season
with the salt, paprika, Worcestershire sauce, Tabasco
and lemon juice. Serve cold.

Iced Coffee

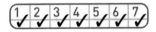

Although this is called iced coffee, it is best not to put ice in it. Just let it get very cold in the fridge. Make sure your coffee is good and strong, as it does lose some of its strength when chilled.

Serves 1

5fl oz (150ml) strong coffee, freshly brewed
5fl oz (150ml) skimmed milk

Mix together and chill.

Darjeeling Cocktail

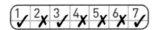

This is an unusual iced tea drink because the tea is infused in cold water. This gives it a much more delicate flavour, making it ideal to serve on a hot day. You could just as well use other types of tea, such as Assam or Lapsang Souchong.

Serves 3

4 pure Darjeeling teabags
1½ pints (845ml) still mineral water, or filtered tap water
1 large orange
a few ice cubes
1 small sprig fresh rosemary
fresh sprigs of mint

Place the teabags in a large jug. Add the cold water, cover, and leave to infuse for 2-3 hours. Stir well, and remove the teabags. Slice the orange, put the ice into the jug, add the orange slices, rosemary and mint, and allow to stand in a cool place for ten minutes before serving.

Hot Milk Toddy

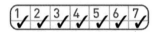

Try and use vanilla extract rather than vanilla essence – it makes a real difference.

Serves 1

8fl oz (220ml) skimmed milk
a few drops vanilla extract
¼ tsp ground nutmeg

Heat the milk and vanilla together. Transfer to a cup and sprinkle the nutmeg on top. Serve hot.

Peach Crush

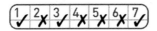

Serves 1

1 large ripe peach
8fl oz (220ml) cold mineral water
crushed ice to serve
mint leaves to garnish

Cut the peach in half, removing the stone, and
liquidise. Put the crushed ice in a glass, top with the
peach purée and fill up with mineral water. Garnish
with the mint leaves.

Strawberry Milk Shake

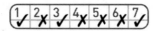

It sounds odd, but a little pepper brings out the flavour of the strawberries.

Serves 1

1 small punnet strawberries
a couple of turns of freshly-ground black pepper
8fl oz (220ml) skimmed milk

Liquidise all the ingredients and serve in a tall glass.

List of Recipes Allowed on Each Day

List of Recipes Allowed on Each Day

The following recipes are listed according to the day you are allowed to eat them. You can then simply choose your daily menu depending on your taste. Remember to bear in mind the maximum allowances for some of the ingredients.

Day One

Cabbage Soup
Bengal Cabbage Soup
Cabbage Soup Italiano
Szechuan Cabbage Soup
Tex-Mex Cabbage Soup

Apple and Blackberry Pie
Baked Apple
Cantaloupe Island
Chinese Gooseberry Salad
Citrus Warmer
Classic Fruit Salad
Darjeeling Cocktail
Florida Cocktail
Fresh Fruit Yoghurt
Grilled Grapefruit
Grilled Orangey Apricots
Grilled Pineapple
Hot Milk Toddy
Hot Ruby Salad
Iced Coffee
Iced Tea with Mint
Melon and Ginger

Peach Crush
Pineapple and Apple
Pineapple and Strawberry Surprise
Salad of Berries
Strawberry Milk Shake
Tangerine Dream
Tropical Fruit Punch
Two of a Kind Pudding

Day Two

Cabbage Soup

Bengal Cabbage Soup
Cabbage Soup Italiano
Szechuan Cabbage Soup
Tex-Mex Cabbage Soup

Artichoke Hearts with Herb Dressing
Asparagus Soup
Asparagus with Yoghurt and Lemon Dressing
Baked Onions
Beetroot with Rosemary
Belgian Salad

Carrots and Artichoke Hearts

Cauliflower Soup

Crudités with a Trio of Dips

Crunchy Jacket Potato

Cucumber and Dill Salad

Cucumber and Mint Soup

Green Asparagus Salad

Green Bean and Savoury Salad

Hot Milk Toddy

Iced Coffee

Iced Tea with Mint

Jacket Potato al Funghi

Jacket Potato with a Garden Salad

Jacket Potato with a Vegetable Medley

Jacket Potato with Baked Vegetables

Jacket Potato with Rosemary

Jacket Potato with Yoghurt and Chives

Minty Jacket Potatoes

Mushroom Soup

Oriental Vegetables

Popeye's Salad

Russian Salad

Sage and Onion Jacket Potato

Spicy Garden Vegetables

Spicy Potato Skins

Welsh Salad

Day Three

Cabbage Soup

Bengal Cabbage Soup
Cabbage Soup Italiano
Szechuan Cabbage Soup
Tex-Mex Cabbage Soup

Apple and Blackberry Pie
Artichoke Hearts with Herb Dressing
Asparagus Soup
Asparagus with Yoghurt and Lemon Dressing
Baked Apple
Baked Onions
Beetroot and Orange Salad
Beetroot with Rosemary
Belgian Salad
Braised Celery with Orange
Cantaloupe Island
Carrots and Artichoke Hearts
Cauliflower Soup
Chinese Gooseberry Salad
Citrus Warmer

Classic Fruit Salad

Crudités with a Trio of Dips

Crunchy Combination Salad

Cucumber and Dill Salad

Cucumber and Mint Soup

Darjeeling Cocktail

Florida Cocktail

Fresh Fruit Yoghurt

Fruity Endive Salad

Green Asparagus Salad

Green Bean and Savoury Salad

Grilled Grapefruit

Grilled Orangey Apricots

Grilled Pineapple

Hot Milk Toddy

Hot Ruby Salad

Iced Coffee

Iced Tea with Mint

Layered Peach, Cucumber and Pepper Salad

Marinated Mushrooms, Apricot and Artichoke Salad

Melon and Ginger

Melon Salad Basket

Melon, Cucumber and Grape Salad

Mushroom Soup

Oriental Vegetables

Peach Crush

Pineapple and Apple

Pineapple and Strawberry Surprise

Popeye's Salad

Russian Salad

Salad of Berries

Spicy Garden Vegetables

Spinach Medley

Strawberry Milk Shake

Tangerine Dream

Tropical Fruit Punch

Two of a Kind Pudding

Welsh Salad

Winter Salad

Day Four

Cabbage Soup

Bengal Cabbage Soup

Cabbage Soup Italiano

Szechuan Cabbage Soup

Tex-Mex Cabbage Soup

Baked Banana

Banana Milk Shake
Banana Whip
Hot Milk Toddy
Iced Coffee
Iced Tea with Mint
Indian Yoghurt Drink

Day Five

Cabbage Soup

Bengal Cabbage Soup
Cabbage Soup Italiano
Szechuan Cabbage Soup
Tex-Mex Cabbage Soup

Chicken and Tomato Kebabs
Chicken en Papillotte
Grilled Trout with Baked Tomatoes
Halibut and Tomato Kebabs
Hot Milk Toddy
Iced Coffee
Iced Tea with Mint
Virgin Mary

Day Six

Cabbage Soup

Bengal Cabbage Soup
Cabbage Soup Italiano
Szechuan Cabbage Soup
Tex-Mex Cabbage Soup

Artichoke Hearts with Herb Dressing
Asparagus Soup
Asparagus with Yoghurt and Lemon Dressing
Baked Fish Italiano
Baked Onions
Beetroot with Rosemary
Belgian Salad
Carrots and Artichoke Hearts
Cauliflower Soup
Chicken and Tomato Kebabs
Chicken Broth
Chicken Curry
Chicken en Papillotte
Chicken in Barbecue Sauce
Cod Steak on a Bed of Vegetable Puree

Crudités with a Trio of Dips

Cucumber and Dill Salad

Cucumber and Mint Soup

English Garden Chicken Salad

Fresh Tuna Kebabs

Gazpacho Salad

Greek Plaki (Fish Soup)

Green Asparagus Salad

Green Bean and Savoury Salad

Grilled Trout with Baked Tomatoes

Haddock en Papillotte

Haddock with Leeks

Halibut and Tomato Kebabs

Hot Milk Toddy

Hot Vegetable Salad

Iced Coffee

Iced Tea with Mint

Mediterranean Chicken Kebabs

Mushroom Soup

Oriental Grilled Fish

Oriental Vegetables

Poached Chicken on a Bed of Three Kinds of

Mushrooms

Popeye's Salad

Russian Chicken Kebabs

Russian Salad

Salade aux Fines Herbes
Sole Roulade
Spicy Garden Vegetables
Stuffed Breast of Chicken
Stuffed Peppers
Tomato and Sorrel Soup
Tomatoes Farcis
Tuna Medley
Virgin Mary
Welsh Salad

Day Seven

Cabbage Soup

Bengal Cabbage Soup
Cabbage Soup Italiano
Szechuan Cabbage Soup
Tex-Mex Cabbage Soup

Apple and Blackberry Pie
Artichoke Hearts with Herb Dressing
Asparagus Soup
Asparagus with Yoghurt and Lemon Dressing

Baked Apple

Baked Onions

Beetroot and Orange Salad

Beetroot with Rosemary

Belgian Salad

Braised Celery with Orange

Cantaloupe Island

Carrots and Artichoke Hearts

Cauliflower Soup

Chinese Gooseberry Salad

Citrus Warmer

Classic Fruit Salad

Crudités with a Trio of Dips

Crunchy Combination Salad

Cucumber and Dill Salad

Cucumber and Mint Soup

Darjeeling Cocktail

Florida Cocktail

Fresh Fruit Yoghurt

Fruity Endive Salad

Green Asparagus Salad

Green Bean and Savoury Salad

Grilled Grapefruit

Grilled Orangey Apricots

Grilled Pineapple

Hot Milk Toddy

Hot Ruby Salad

Iced Coffee

Iced Tea with Mint

Layered Peach, Cucumber and Pepper Salad

Marinated Mushroom, Apricot and Artichoke Salad

Melon and Ginger

Melon Salad Basked

Melon, Cucumber and Grape Salad

Mushroom Soup

Oriental Vegetables

Peach Crush

Pineapple and Apple

Pineapple and Strawberry Surprise

Popeye's Salad

Russian Salad

Salad of Berries

Spicy Garden Vegetables

Spinach Medley

Strawberry Milk Shake

Tangerine Dream

Tropical Fruit Punch

Two of a Kind Pudding

Welsh Salad

Winter Salad

Two Weekly Menus

Two Weekly Menus

Here are two sample weekly menus to help your choose what to eat over your seven-day diet. You can either follow these exactly, adapt them, or invent your own.

If you decide to adapt them or invent your own, remember to follow these golden rules:

1. Make sure that you are using a dish that is allowed on a particular day. Each recipe indicates which day it is allowed.
2. Make sure you are not exceeding your allowed quantities of restricted ingredients. For example, if you have a recipe for lunch that includes 8fl oz natural yoghurt, you can't have anything for dinner that includes yoghurt. Or if, on day 2, you have a jacket potato for dinner, you can't have one for lunch.
3. Remember that on any one particular day, you can have either yoghurt or milk. You can't mix the two.

As long as you follow these simple rules, you will be able to create hundreds of delicious menus.

Menu 1

DAY 1

Breakfast
Citrus Warmer (p.102)
&
Tropical Fruit Punch (p.148)

Lunch
Bengal Cabbage Soup (p.28)
&
Apple and Blackberry Pie (p.114)

Dinner
Cabbage Soup (p.19)
&
Pineapple and Strawberry Surprise
(p.110)
&
Hot Milk Toddy (p.152)

DAY 2

Breakfast
Crudites with a Trio of Dips (p.88)
&
Hot Milk Toddy (p.152)

Lunch
Tex-Mex Cabbage Soup (p.36)
&
Baked Onions (p.77)
&
Oriental Vegetables (p.72)

Dinner
Cabbage Soup (p.19)
&
Minty Jacket Potato (p.138)
&
Popeye's Salad (p.86)

DAY 3

Breakfast
Florida Cocktail (p.108)

Lunch
Cabbage Soup (p.19)
&
Green Asparagus Salad (p.85)
&
Fruity Endive Salad (p.128)
&
Hot Ruby Salad (p.101)

Dinner
Cabbage Soup (p.19)
&
Green Bean and Savoury Salad (p.69)
&
Remainder of Day's Allowance of
Yoghurt, with a piece of Fresh Free
Fruit

DAY 4

Breakfast
Banana Milk Shake (p.145)

Lunch
Cabbage Soup (p.19)
&
Banana Whip (p.111)
&
16fl oz (440ml) Skimmed Milk

Afternoon
16fl oz (440ml) Skimmed Milk

Dinner
Cabbage Soup (p.19)
&
2–3 Baked Bananas served with 4fl oz
(110ml) Yoghurt (p.96)
&
16fl oz (440ml) Hot Milk Toddy
(p.152)

DAY 5

Breakfast
Grilled Trout with Baked Tomatoes
(p.55)

Lunch
Cabbage Soup (p.19)

Dinner
Cabbage Soup (p.19)
&
Chicken en Papillotte (p.39)
&
8fl oz (220ml) Hot Milk Toddy (p.152)

DAY 6

Breakfast
Gazpacho Salad (p.82)

Lunch
Cabbage Soup (p.19)
&
English Garden Chicken Salad (p.46)
&
Greek Plaki (p.31)

Dinner
Cabbage Soup (p.19)
&
Fresh Tuna Kebabs (p.61)
&
Russian Chicken Kebabs (p.51)
&
4fl oz (110ml) Low-Fat Natural
Yoghurt

Day 7

Breakfast
Cantaloupe Island (p.115)

Lunch
Cabbage Soup (p.19)
&
Pineapple and Apple (p.104)
&
Oriental Vegetables (p.72)
&
Tropical Fruit Punch (p.148)

Dinner
Cabbage Soup (p.19)
&
Winter Salad (p.120)
&
Braised Celery with Orange (p.122)
&
Strawberry Milk Shake (p.154)

Menu 2

DAY 1

Breakfast
Fresh Fruit Yoghurt (p.113)
&
Grilled Grapefruit (p.98)

Lunch
Szechuan Cabbage Soup (p.26)
&
Chinese Gooseberry Salad (p.107)
&
Iced Tea with Mint (p.146)

Dinner
Cabbage Soup (p.19)
&
Two of a Kind Pudding (p.97)

DAY 2

Breakfast
Cabbage Soup (p.19)

Lunch
Cabbage Soup (p.19)
&
Jacket Potato with Baked Vegetables
(p.141)

Dinner
Cucumber and Mint Soup (p.33)
&
Russian Salad (p.90)

DAY 3

Breakfast
Classic Fruit Salad (p.116)

Lunch
Cabbage Soup (p.19)
&
Beetroot with Rosemary (p.70)
&
Spicy Garden Vegetables (p.73)
&
Baked Apple (p.95)

Dinner
Cabbage Soup (p.19)
&
Marinated Mushroom, Apricot and
Artichoke Salad (p.124)
&
Grilled Pineapple (p.100)
&
Peach Crush (p.153)

DAY 4

Breakfast
2-3 Baked Bananas (p.96)
&
16fl oz (440ml) Hot Milk Toddy
(p.152)

Lunch
Cabbage Soup (p.19)
&
2 bananas
&
Indian Yoghurt Drink (p.147)

Afternoon
16fl oz (440ml) Skimmed Milk or Hot
Milk Toddy (p.152)

Dinner
Cabbage Soup (p.19)
&
Banana Milk Shake (p.145)
&
8fl oz (220ml) Hot Milk Toddy (p.152)

Day 5

Breakfast
Cabbage Soup (p.19)

Lunch
Cabbage Soup (p.19)
&
Chicken and Tomato Kebabs (p.40)

Dinner
Grilled Trout with Baked Tomatoes
(p.55)
&
8fl oz (220ml) Hot Milk Toddy
(p.152)

Day 6

Breakfast
Tuna Medley (p.57)

Lunch
Cabbage Soup (p.19)
&
Sole Roulade (p. 58)
&
Cucumber and Dill Salad (p.81)
&
Mediterranean Chicken Kebabs (p.52)

Dinner
Cabbage Soup (p.19)
&
Stuffed Breast of Chicken (p.42)
&
Baked Fish Italiano (p.62)
&
Salade aux Fines Herbes (p.84)
&
Remainder of the Daily Allowance
Yoghurt

DAY 7

Breakfast
Tangerine Dream (p.103)

Lunch
Cabbage Soup (p.19)
&
Melon and Ginger (p.109)
&
Asparagus with Yoghurt and Lemon
Dressing (p.75)
&
3fl oz (75ml) yoghurt with a piece of
free fruit
&
Tropical Fruit Punch (p.148)

Dinner
Cabbage Soup (p.19)
&
Baked Onions (p.77)
&
Beetroot and Orange Salad (p.123)
&
Spinach Medley (p.126)
&
Classic Fruit Salad (p.116)

The
Ingredients
Table

How to Use the Ingredients Table

This table details exactly what you can eat on which day. Sometimes it is difficult to keep track of what you have eaten, which is where this table comes in so useful. You should photocopy this table so that you can re-use it whenever you want to do the diet. Here are a couple of examples of how to use it.

Example 1
On day 4 you have a double-quantity Banana Milk Shake (p.) for breakfast. This involves 16fl oz skimmed milk and 2 bananas. On the day 4 column, you should therefore tick off two of the 8s in the skimmed milk row, and tick off the 1 and the 2 in the banana row. At a glance, you will then see that you have 6 x 8fl oz portions of milk left, and 4 bananas. You could choose to substitute one of the remaining 8fl oz portions of milk for an 8fl oz portion of low-fat yoghurt.

Example 2
On day 5 you have Grilled Trout with Baked Tomatoes (p.) for lunch. This involves two tomatoes, so you should therefore tick off the 1 and the 2 in the tomato row. At a glance you can then see that you have four tomatoes left to eat on that day.

	DAY 1				DAY 2				DAY 3			
CABBAGE SOUP	Unlimited				Unlimited				Unlimited			
FREE FRUITS	Unlimited								Unlimited			
FREE VEGETABLES					Unlimited				Unlimited			
LOW-FAT YOGHURT * OR	1	2	3	4	1	2	3	4	1	2	3	4
SKIMMED MILK (fl oz)	5	6	7	8	5	6	7	8	5	6	7	8
LOW-CALORIE DRESSING	1 tbsp				1 tbsp				1 tbsp			
BANANAS												
JACKET POTATO					1 large jacket potato							
FISH												
CHICKEN												
TOMATOES												

* Remember, you cannot mix low-fat yoghurt or skimmed milk in one day, except on day 4, when you can choose to substitute one of your 8x8fl oz skimmed

DAY 4				DAY 5				DAY 6				DAY 7			
Unlimited				Unlimited				Unlimited				Unlimited			
												Unlimited			
								Unlimited				Unlimited			
8	8	8	8	1	2	3	4	1	2	3	4	1	2	3	4
8	8	8	8	5	6	7	8	5	6	7	8	5	6	7	8
1 tbsp				1 tbsp				1 tbsp				1 tbsp			
1	2	3													
4	5	6													
				Unlimited				Unlimited							
				Unlimited				Unlimited							
				1	2	3		Unlimited							
				4	5	6									

milk with 1x8fl oz low-fat yoghurt. Make a photocopy of this page and keep track of the total number of fluid ounces you consume by marking off the relevant box.

Index of
Recipes

Index of Recipes